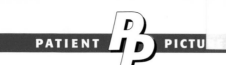 

PATIENT **PP** PICTU

Clinical drawings for your patients

Gynaecological oncology

by Andy Nordin MBBS MRCOG
Senior Registrar and Oncology Fellow,
Gynaecological Oncology Centre,
Queen Elizabeth Hospital, Gateshead, Tyne and Wear, UK

Series Editor: J Richard Smith MD MRCOG
Consultant Gynaecologist, Chelsea and
Westminster Hospital, London, UK,
and Honorary Consultant Gynaecologist,
Royal Brompton Hospital, London, UK

Illustrated by Dee McLean, MeDee Art, London, UK

D1297436

Patient Pictures – Gynaecological oncology

Text © Andy Nordin 1999
Health Press Limited, Elizabeth House, Queen Street,
Abingdon, Oxford OX14 3JR, UK
Tel: +44 (0)1235 523233
Fax: +44 (0)1235 523238

Patient Pictures is a trade mark of Health Press Limited.

The publisher and the author have made every effort to
ensure the accuracy of this book, but cannot accept
responsibility for any errors or omissions.

A CIP catalogue record for this title is available from the
British Library.

ISBN 1-899541-21-7

Printed by The Ethedo Press Limited, High Wycombe, UK.

Reproduction authorization

The purchaser of this *Patient Pictures* series title is hereby authorized to reproduce by photocopy only, any part of the pictorial and textual material contained in this work for non-profit, educational, or patient education use. Photocopying for these purposes only is welcomed and free from further permission requirements from the publisher and free from any fee.

The reproduction of any material from this publication outside the guidelines above is strictly prohibited without the permission in writing of the publisher and is subject to minimum charges laid down by the Publishers Licensing Society Limited or its nominees.

Sarah Redston

Publisher, Health Press Limited, Oxford

Author's preface

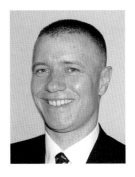

Over 15 000 women in the UK are diagnosed with cancer of the genital tract every year. While gynaecological cancers still cause great suffering and claim many lives, earlier diagnosis of disease, new and refined surgical techniques, and progress in radiotherapy, chemotherapy and palliation management mean that patients have a better prognosis and quality of life than ever before.

The diagnosis of cancer makes patients anxious and uncertain about their future. I believe that providing honest and reliable information helps women at this time of crisis. It enables them to become active participants in management decisions that carry profound implications for their quality of life. This book is designed as an information resource for patients and their families, and as a counselling aid for healthcare professionals. The pages are designed for easy photocopying so that the appropriate information can be given to the patient and/or carer to take home. I hope it will be used to help empower women to make informed choices for themselves.

Andy Nordin MBBS MRCOG
Queen Elizabeth Hospital, Gateshead, Tyne and Wear, UK

The female genital tract

- The female genital tract includes the vulva, vagina, cervix, uterus, Fallopian tubes and ovaries.

- The vulva is the area surrounding the openings of the vagina and urethra. It includes the clitoris.

- The vagina is a muscular tube that runs from the vulva to the cervix.

- The cervix, which is sometimes called the neck of the womb, is quite firm and lies at the bottom of the uterus. During labour, it softens and then opens to allow the baby to be born.

- The uterus is a muscular organ, usually about the size of a pear, that sits in the pelvis. It is here that the fetus develops during pregnancy. The lining of the uterus is called the endometrium. This thickens during the menstrual cycle in preparation for a fertilized egg, and is shed during menstruation if the egg is not fertilized.

- The two ovaries sit on either side of the uterus. As well as producing eggs, they produce the female hormones, oestrogen and progesterone, until the menopause occurs.

- The Fallopian tubes connect the uterus to the ovaries. When an egg is released from one of the ovaries, it is collected by the Fallopian tube. Once in the tube, it may be fertilized by a sperm that has swum up from the vagina through the cervix and uterus.

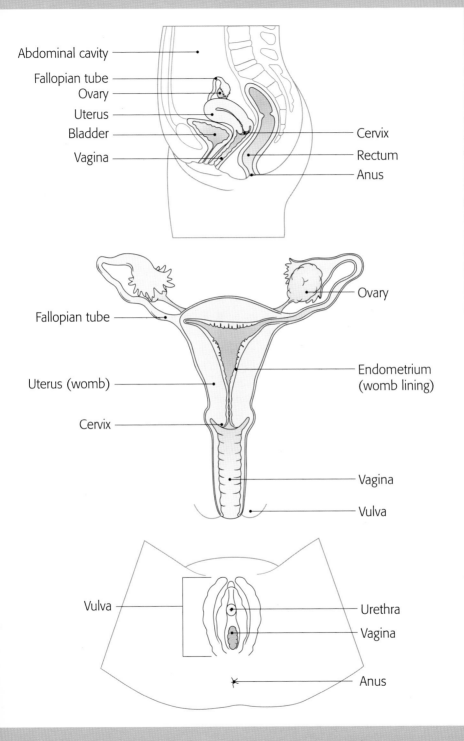

The lymphatic system

- Lymph vessels are very fine tubes that drain the fluid, called lymph, which escapes into the body's tissues. They run next to the arteries and form a network that returns the watery fluid into the bloodstream near the heart.

- Lymph nodes, sometimes called glands, are swellings that occur near to the main arteries. They act as filters for the lymph, and also have a role in the body's immune system.

- Microscopic cancer cells can escape into lymph, and can become trapped in lymph nodes. If the cells then grow, they form growths called metastases. This is one of the common ways that many cancers can spread to different parts of the body.

- Surgery for many types of cancer (including cervical, endometrial and vulval cancers) usually involves removing lymph nodes and the nearby lymph vessels.

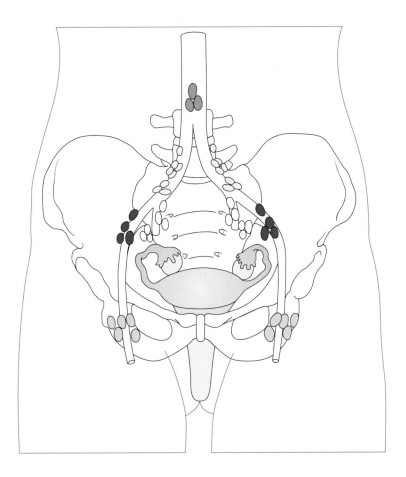

 Para-aortic nodes

 Common iliac nodes

 Internal iliac and obturator nodes

 External iliac nodes

 Inguinal (groin) nodes

Pelvic and groin lymph nodes

- Cervical intraepithelial neoplasia (CIN for short) is a pre-cancerous change in the part of the cervix that juts into the vagina. This area, where the skin lining the cervix changes to the glandular lining of the cervical canal, is called the 'transformation zone'.

- A smear test that shows abnormal cells ('dyskaryosis') means CIN may be present on the cervix. Your gynaecologist will examine the cervix with a special microscope called a colposcope. If CIN is present, certain changes in the skin over the cervix show up after applying a dilute vinegar solution. CIN can only be diagnosed by taking a sample of tissue (a biopsy) from the cervix for microscopic examination.

- CIN is graded as 1, 2 or 3, depending on how the tissue looks under a microscope. Even CIN 3 is not cancer and is easily treated. However, if CIN 2 or 3 is not treated, there is a risk that cancer will develop. CIN 2 and 3 are called high-grade CIN.

- CIN 1 (low-grade CIN) is a minor pre-cancerous change that often goes away without treatment. It is not usually necessary to treat (remove or destroy) CIN 1 at first diagnosis. However, in some women, it slowly progresses to high-grade CIN.

- If you have CIN 1, it is very important to monitor your cervix with colposcopy and smear tests every 6 months or so. If the CIN 1 does not go away after 1–2 years, you may be offered treatment. If high-grade CIN (CIN 2 or 3) develops, you will definitely need treatment.

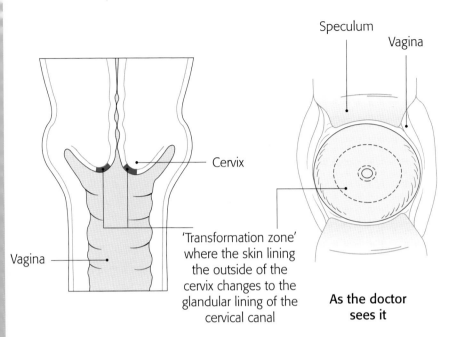

Speculum

Vagina

Cervix

Vagina

'Transformation zone'
where the skin lining
the outside of the
cervix changes to the
glandular lining of the
cervical canal

**As the doctor
sees it**

Development of CIN and cervical cancer

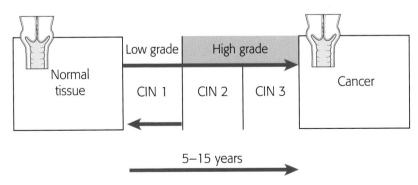

Normal tissue

Low grade | High grade

CIN 1 | CIN 2 | CIN 3

Cancer

5–15 years

Cervical cancer

- There are two main types of cervical cancer. The first type grows in the skin lining the cervix. The second type grows from the lining of the mucous glands of the cervix. Most cervical cancers are associated with infection by a virus called a wart virus.

- Cervical cancer has two main ways of spreading: local invasion and lymphatic spread. The spread of cancer to different parts of the body is called metastasis.

- Local invasion means that the tumour grows into the upper vagina, the uterus and the tissue in the pelvis next to the uterus. In advanced cancer, the tumour may grow into the bladder at the front of the cervix and into the rectum at the back. It may also block the ureters, the tubes that carry urine from the kidneys to the bladder, causing kidney failure.

- Lymphatic spread occurs when cancerous cells move through the lymph fluid channels and are trapped by lymph glands, where the cells can multiply and form tumours.

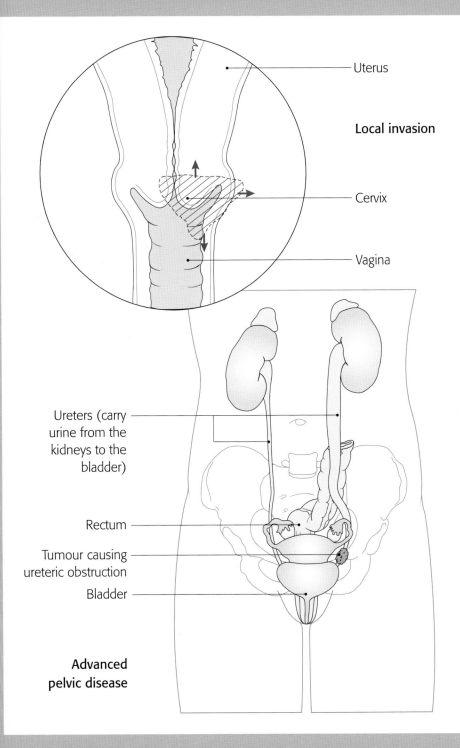

Uterus

Local invasion

Cervix

Vagina

Ureters (carry
urine from the
kidneys to the
bladder)

Rectum

Tumour causing
ureteric obstruction

Bladder

**Advanced
pelvic disease**

Cervical smear

- The cervical smear test is carried out to look for a change in the skin lining the part of the cervix that juts into the vagina. Such a change is described as 'pre-cancerous'. It is not cancer, but it does indicate that cancer may develop if the condition remains untreated.

- For a smear test, you will be asked to lie on your back with your legs bent and your knees parted. A plastic or metal instrument, called a speculum, is inserted into the vagina to hold it open so that the cervix can be seen.

- The doctor or nurse will examine the cervix and collect some cervical cells. This is done by gently scraping the cervix in a circular motion using a specially designed spatula and possibly also a small brush. The cells are smeared onto a glass slide, and will be examined under a microscope in the laboratory.

- A smear test only takes a few minutes. It is not painful but can be a bit uncomfortable.

- Your doctor or nurse will be able to tell you how long it will take to get the test results.

- The abnormal appearance of cells on a smear associated with pre-cancerous changes is called dyskaryosis.

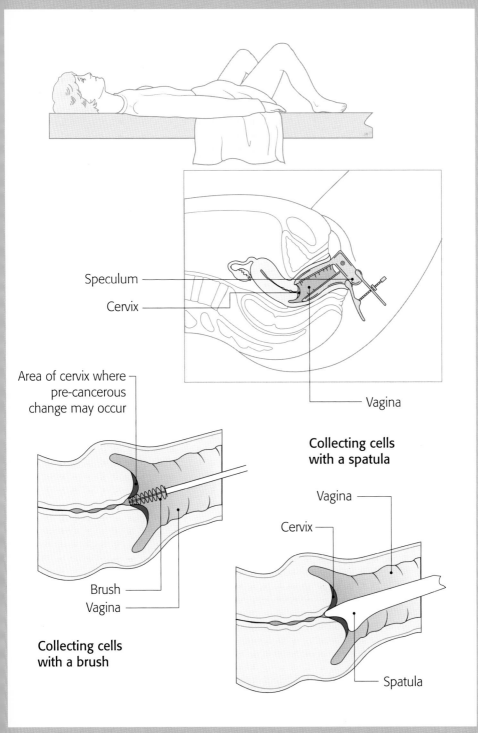

Speculum

Cervix

Vagina

Collecting cells with a spatula

Area of cervix where pre-cancerous change may occur

Brush

Vagina

Collecting cells with a brush

Vagina

Cervix

Spatula

Colposcopy and treatment of abnormal smear

- Colposcopy is carried out if the smear test shows up abnormalities in the cervical cells. A colposcope is a microscope that magnifies the cervix.

- Colposcopy is a painless, out-patient procedure. You will be asked to lie on your back with your legs in supports.

- A plastic or metal instrument called a speculum is inserted into the vagina to hold the walls of the vagina apart. The speculum is similar to that used for a smear.

- Dilute acetic acid, and possibly iodine, will be painted onto your cervix to show up any abnormalities. Small samples of tissue, called biopsies, may be taken from the cervix and sent to the laboratory for analysis. These procedures do not hurt but may be a bit uncomfortable.

- During colposcopy, abnormal cervical cells can be removed or destroyed in a number of ways. The most common is called loop biopsy or LLETZ. A local anaesthetic is injected to numb your cervix. This is not painful but may be uncomfortable. A small piece of tissue containing the abnormal cells is then removed using an electrical current; the sample removed is about the size of a marble. Other methods involve heating or freezing the area with the abnormal cells, or removing or destroying it using a laser.

- You are likely to have discharge and abnormal bleeding for a few weeks after treatment. If the bleeding is heavy or if the discharge becomes offensive, consult your doctor.

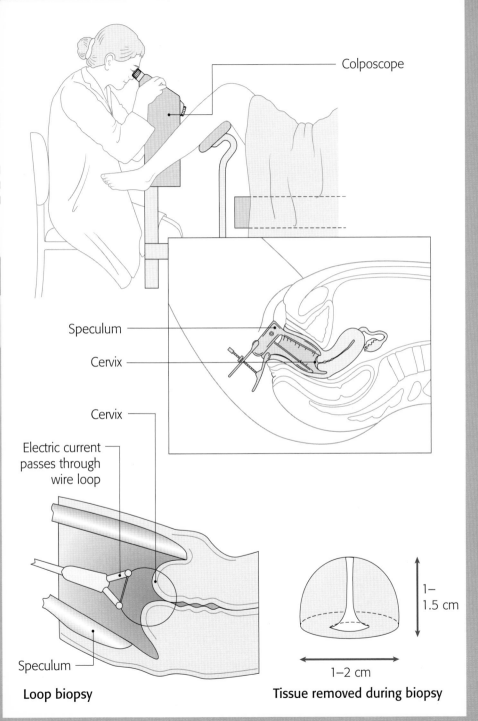

Colposcope

Speculum

Cervix

Cervix

Electric current
passes through
wire loop

Speculum

Loop biopsy

1–
1.5 cm

1–2 cm

Tissue removed during biopsy

Cystoscopy, biopsy and sigmoidoscopy

- Treatment of cervical cancer depends on the stage that the disease has reached. This is a measure of the size of the tumour and how far it has spread. Your doctor may carry out several different investigations (including a thorough pelvic examination), often under general anaesthetic.

- A piece of tissue, called a biopsy, may be removed in the colposcopy clinic or while you are anaesthetized. This is then sent to the laboratory for analysis.

- Your bladder may be examined in a procedure called cystoscopy. A narrow telescope, called a cystoscope, is inserted into your urethra, to examine the bladder for signs that it has been affected by the cancer. The urethra is the tube through which urine passes out of the body.

- The lower part of the bowel may be examined in a procedure called sigmoidoscopy. A metal or plastic tube, called a sigmoidoscope, is inserted into the back passage.

- After these investigations, you may feel some discomfort when you go to the toilet, but this should pass within a day or so.

- Many patients with cervical cancer do not need these investigations.

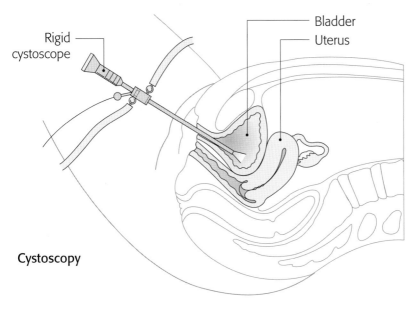

Rigid cystoscope

Bladder

Uterus

Cystoscopy

Sigmoidoscopy

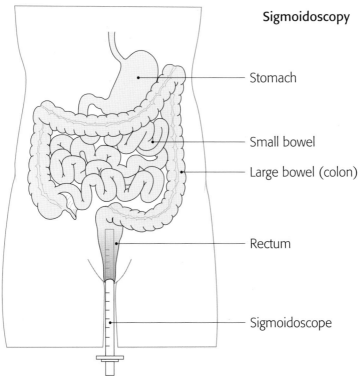

Stomach

Small bowel

Large bowel (colon)

Rectum

Sigmoidoscope

Imaging investigations: IVU, CT and MRI

- Radiological investigations can be used to find out how large a cancer is and how far it has spread.

- An intravenous urogram (IVU for short) uses dye to show up the kidneys and ureters, which can then be seen on X-ray. The dye is injected through a vein in the back of your hand.

- The hospital will give you any special instructions – these may include not eating or drinking anything for 6 hours before the test, and possibly using a laxative on the day before the procedure, to help to clear your bowels.

- With CT (computerized tomography) scans, X-rays of the abdomen and pelvis are taken in sequence to build up a picture of the whole area, rather like slices through a loaf of bread.

- You may be asked to have a special drink of 'dye' before your scan. The scan may also be repeated after you have had some dye injected into the vein in the back of your hand. This helps to show up blood vessels on the scan.

- MRI stands for magnetic resonance imaging and uses a magnetic field to scan the abdomen and build up an image. There are no X-rays involved in this procedure.

- Having a CT or, particularly, an MRI scan can be claustrophobic and noisy, but it is not at all painful. The hospital will let you know if you need to make any particular preparations before your scan.

MRI

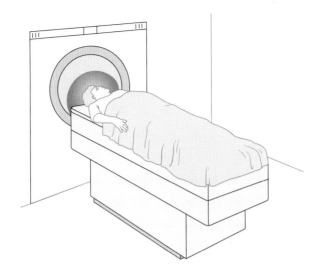

CT

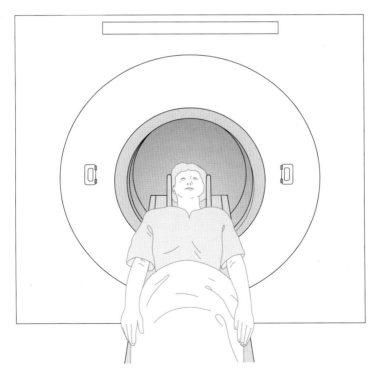

Loop biopsy, cone biopsy and simple hysterectomy

- If a cervical cancer is at a very early stage, it may be possible to treat it by removing just the lower part of the cervix. This may be performed using an electrical current (or diathermy) in a procedure known as loop biopsy, or a laser or a knife, in a cone biopsy. It may be carried out using a local or a general anaesthetic.

- You are likely to notice some discharge and abnormal bleeding afterwards, and this may continue for several weeks. Although you can get back to normal the day after the operation, you need to give your cervix time to heal. Avoid using tampons, and do not have penetrative sex for 4 weeks. If the bleeding is heavy or the discharge becomes offensive, see your doctor.

- Occasionally, women are advised to have a 'simple' hysterectomy, where the uterus and cervix are removed under general anaesthetic. However, this is a rare treatment for cervical cancer.

- Following simple hysterectomy, a catheter may be passed up the urethra into the bladder to drain off the urine, and another tube may drain any bleeding from your abdomen. These tubes may be left in place for 1–2 days.

- Afterwards, you will be given painkillers. Any non-dissolvable skin stitches or staples will be removed after 5–7 days, before you go home. After 6 weeks, your vagina will have healed fully, and will function normally.

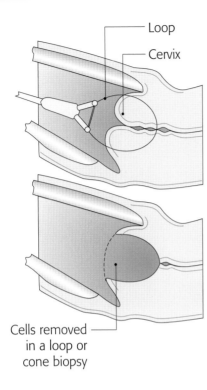

Loop

Cervix

Cells removed in a loop or cone biopsy

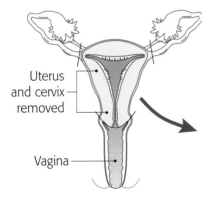

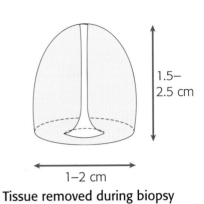

1.5–2.5 cm

1–2 cm

Tissue removed during biopsy

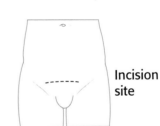

Incision site

Uterus and cervix removed

Vagina

'Simple' hysterectomy

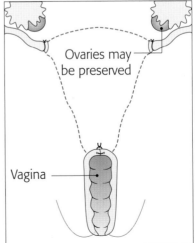

Ovaries may be preserved

Vagina

Radical hysterectomy

- Radical hysterectomy, sometimes called Wertheim's hysterectomy, is performed for cancer of the cervix. Advanced stages of this cancer are best treated by radiotherapy (X-ray treatment) and chemotherapy.

- Radical hysterectomy involves removing the uterus, Fallopian tubes, cervix, the very top part of the vagina, lymph glands in the pelvis and, sometimes, the ovaries. The vagina may be shortened as a result.

- During the operation, a catheter is passed either up through the urethra or through the abdomen and into the bladder, to drain off the urine. You may have another tube in your abdomen or vagina to drain any slight bleeding. The catheter is usually left in for at least 5 days, and the other tube is usually left in place for 1–2 days. It sometimes takes several weeks before your bladder begins to work properly again, and changes in bladder sensation and function are sometimes permanent.

- You will be given painkillers to relieve the pain after the operation. Because your ovaries make the female hormones oestrogen and progesterone, you may also be prescribed hormone-replacement therapy (HRT), if your ovaries have been removed.

- A course of radiotherapy and chemotherapy may be necessary after surgery.

- After the operation, avoid having penetrative sex for about 6 weeks to allow the top of the vagina to heal fully.

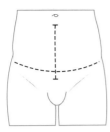

Incision sites

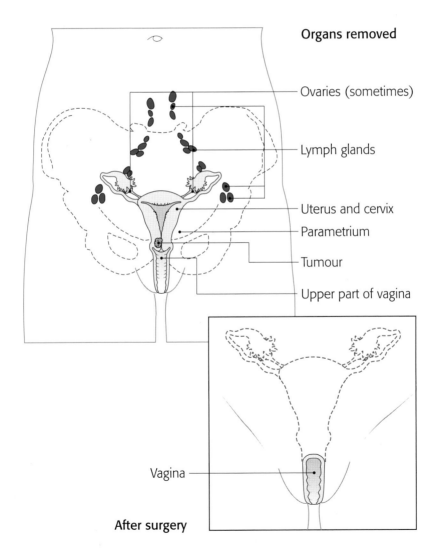

Organs removed

Ovaries (sometimes)

Lymph glands

Uterus and cervix

Parametrium

Tumour

Upper part of vagina

Vagina

After surgery

Laparoscopically assisted radical vaginal hysterectomy and radical trachelectomy

- Laparoscopically assisted radical vaginal hysterectomy and radical trachelectomy are newer alternatives to radical hysterectomy. Performed only in certain specialist centres, they are only suitable for small cancers. They are carried out under general anaesthetic.

- For these keyhole surgery procedures, a small cut is made in the belly button and the abdomen is filled with gas. A narrow telescope, called a laparoscope, is then inserted so that the surgeon can see into the abdomen. Various keyhole surgery instruments are passed through other small cuts in the abdomen wall. The surgeon removes the lymph glands in the pelvis through the small cuts.

- In a laparoscopically assisted radical vaginal hysterectomy, the uterus, Fallopian tubes and, sometimes but not always, ovaries are initially freed from their attachments using the laparoscope. The uterus and its surrounding tissue, the cervix and the top part of the vagina are finally removed through the vagina.

- In radical trachelectomy, the cervix and upper part of the vagina are removed, but the uterus is left in place. The lymph glands in the pelvis are also removed, usually by keyhole surgery. This is only suitable for tumours caught in the early stage. As the uterus is left in place, you can, potentially, still become pregnant. A stitch is made at the bottom of the uterus, and this takes the place of the cervix in supporting a pregnancy. A baby would be delivered by Caesarean section.

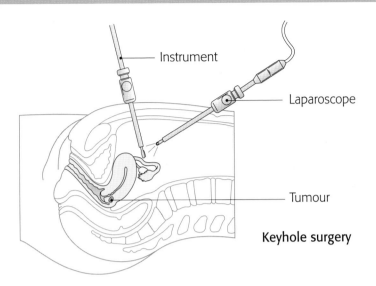

Instrument

Laparoscope

Tumour

Keyhole surgery

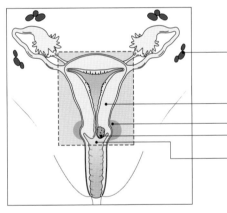

Radical vaginal hysterectomy

Lymph glands removed
using keyhole surgery

Uterus

Parametrium

Tumour

Upper vagina

Organs
removed
vaginally

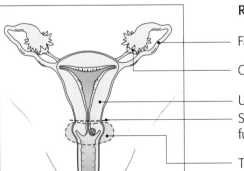

Radical trachelectomy

Fallopian tube

Ovary

Uterus

Stitch to support
future pregnancy

Tissue removed

Vagina

Ovarian cancer

- There are many different types of ovarian cancer, corresponding with the different types of cells in the ovary. The most common group result from abnormal growth of the 'skin' of the ovary. Other types grow from the tissue that surrounds the eggs in the ovary, and the egg cells can also become cancerous.

- Ovarian cysts and lumps can be benign, meaning that they are not cancerous. Other types of cysts and lumps grow very slowly over a long period of time. These are classified as borderline tumours of low malignant potential. The exact diagnosis may not be known until after the ovaries have been examined under the microscope after surgery.

- Cancer of the ovary can occur in one or both ovaries. It spreads directly to other organs in the pelvis, such as the Fallopian tubes and the uterus. The tumours also produce a fluid called ascites, and cells in the ascites can spread the cancer to the lining of the abdomen (the peritoneum), the bowel and other organs. An 'apron' of fat inside the abdomen, called the omentum, is also often involved. The tumours can block the bowel, causing vomiting and weight loss. It may also spread to the chest, causing problems with breathing.

Stage I	Cancer confined to ovaries 1a: one ovary 1b: both ovaries 1c: on or through the surface of the ovary or in ascitic fluid or washings of the abdomen
Stage II	Spread within pelvis only
Stage III	Spread into abdomen or to lymph glands in pelvis or groins
Stage IV	Spread beyond abdomen and pelvis (e.g. to chest) or within liver

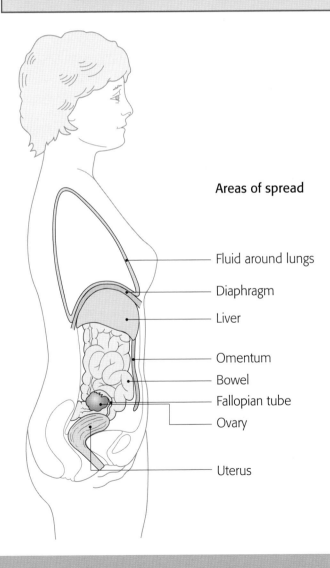

Areas of spread

Fluid around lungs

Diaphragm

Liver

Omentum

Bowel

Fallopian tube

Ovary

Uterus

Ultrasound and Ca125

- Before you have surgery for ovarian cancer, you may have an ultrasound scan. Your abdomen is coated with jelly, and the probe is moved smoothly across it. Harmless, high-frequency sound waves from the probe build an image on a television screen. A probe can also be used in the vagina to give a clear picture of the uterus and ovaries. Both of these types of scan are painless.

- You may have a chest X-ray before surgery. You may also have an MRI or CT scan to give the surgeon detailed pictures of the liver, lymph glands and other abdominal organs.

- Before surgery, a blood sample is taken to check your blood cell counts, blood group, and that your liver and kidneys are working properly.

- A protein called Ca125 will also be measured in the blood sample. Ca125 is a tumour marker, which means that the level of it in your blood may get higher as the cancer becomes more advanced. If your Ca125 level is raised, this marker may be used to monitor the response of your cancer to treatment, and to look for return of the disease.

- Ca125 and ultrasound are being investigated as screening tests for early ovarian cancer, particularly for women with a strong family history.

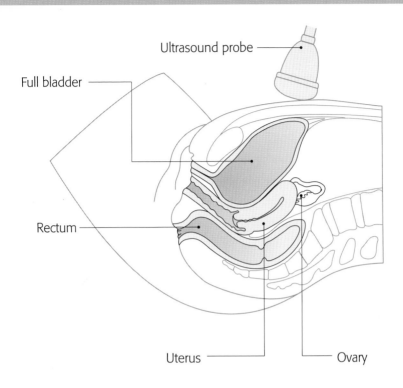

Ultrasound probe

Full bladder

Rectum

Uterus

Ovary

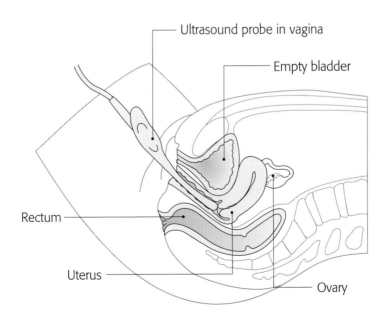

Ultrasound probe in vagina

Empty bladder

Rectum

Uterus

Ovary

TAH & BSO and omentectomy, and debulking surgery

- If your ovarian cancer is at an early stage, you will probably have a total abdominal hysterectomy and bilateral salpingo-oophorectomy (TAH & BSO). This involves removing the uterus, cervix, Fallopian tubes and ovaries. The pelvic lymph glands may also be removed. The fat 'apron' in the abdomen (the omentum) is also removed in a procedure called omentectomy.

- The operation is carried out under general anaesthetic. A catheter will drain urine from the bladder for a few days, and you will stay in hospital for about 1 week.

- Your doctor may not know whether your tumour is benign or cancerous or, if cancerous, how advanced it is, until the pathology report is available, usually 3–7 days after the operation.

- If the cancer is advanced, it is necessary to remove as much of the tumour as possible during the operation; this is called debulking surgery, and may involve bowel surgery. This does not cure ovarian cancer, but can delay or prevent complications such as bowel or kidney obstruction. It also makes chemotherapy, which is treatment with drugs that attack the cancer cells, more effective.

- If the cancer affects only one ovary, and you have yet to complete your family, a unilateral oophorectomy may be an option. This involves removing only the affected ovary. You may be recommended to have the other ovary removed with a hysterectomy later.

Incision site

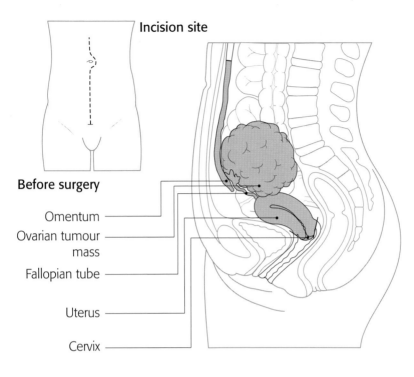

Before surgery

Omentum

Ovarian tumour
mass

Fallopian tube

Uterus

Cervix

After surgery

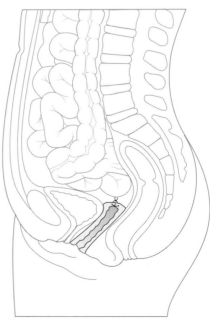

Chemotherapy

- Chemotherapy is treatment with drugs that destroy cancer cells. If the cancer has spread beyond your ovary, you will probably be given chemotherapy after surgery. Sometimes, chemotherapy is given before surgery if your doctor thinks that you are not strong enough to have an operation when your cancer is first diagnosed.

- Chemotherapy drugs are also poisonous to normal cells, and might cause side-effects such as temporary hair loss. Blood cells are also damaged, so you may need blood transfusions and drugs to stop infections. Chemotherapy is given in 'cycles' to allow your normal cells to recover between treatments. Chemotherapy may make you feel sick, but there are effective anti-sickness drugs that can prevent this.

- New chemotherapy drugs and combinations are constantly being developed and tested. Currently, the majority of patients are offered carboplatin together with paclitaxel (Taxol®). Some patients are suitable to receive carboplatin alone.

- It is usual for chemotherapy to be given by a drip every 3 weeks for six treatments. If the cancer returns or does not respond to the chemotherapy, other treatments may be effective.

- Your specialist and chemotherapy nurses will tell you about your treatment and the specific side-effects that you might expect.

Chemotherapy

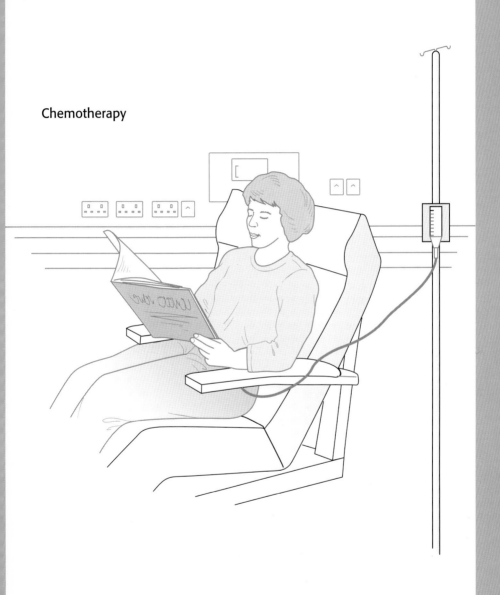

Endometrial cancer

- The endometrium is the tissue that lines the uterus. Endometrial cancer usually occurs in women after the menopause, causing vaginal bleeding, though it can occur before the menopause, causing bleeding between periods.

- Endometrial cancer is often triggered by a hormone imbalance. Hormones are the chemical messengers that regulate the body's functions. Women have two main reproductive hormones, called oestrogen and progesterone. Progesterone, the hormone released when a woman ovulates, helps to protect against endometrial cancer. Progesterone is also present in hormonal contraceptives including the pill.

- A pre-cancerous form exists, called atypical endometrial hyperplasia. Depending on how abnormal the cells are, this can be treated with progesterone therapy or hysterectomy.

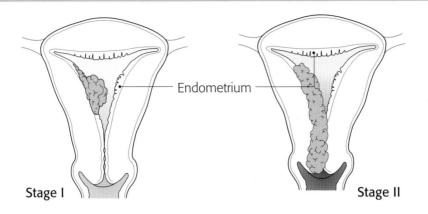

Endometrium

Stage I

Stage II

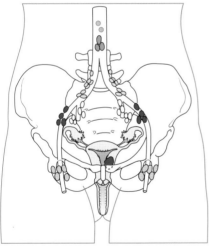

Stage III

Any of:
- outer surface of uterus
- Fallopian tube or ovary
- pelvic/para-aortic lymph nodes

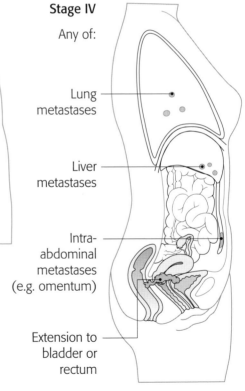

Stage IV

Any of:

Lung metastases

Liver metastases

Intra-abdominal metastases (e.g. omentum)

Extension to bladder or rectum

Endometrial biopsy and ultrasound

- Endometrial biopsy and ultrasound can both be used to investigate the cause of abnormal bleeding.

- An endometrial biopsy is a sample of tissue taken from the lining of the uterus, known as the endometrium. The biopsy is usually carried out as an out-patient procedure without an anaesthetic.

- You will be asked to lie on your back with your legs apart. A plastic or metal instrument called a speculum is inserted into the vagina to hold the vaginal walls apart. A narrow plastic device is then passed into the vagina, through the cervix and into the uterus, where it is used to remove a piece of tissue. This is then sent to the laboratory.

- Endometrial biopsy is not usually painful. If you have not been pregnant, however, your cervix might be tightly closed. If this is the case, local anaesthetic can be used to numb the cervix, and a metal instrument can be used to open it gently. Sometimes a general anaesthetic is needed.

- You can get back to normal straight away after an endometrial biopsy, but you may have spotting of blood for a few days afterwards. Laboratory results should be with your doctor in about a week.

- With ultrasound, a probe is gently placed in the vagina, and the image of the uterus is seen on a screen. Scan results are available immediately, but you may have to wait for your doctor to interpret them and inform you.

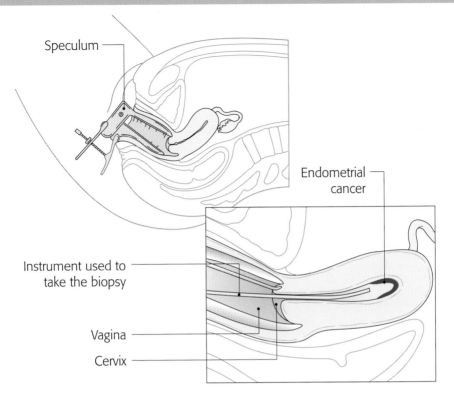

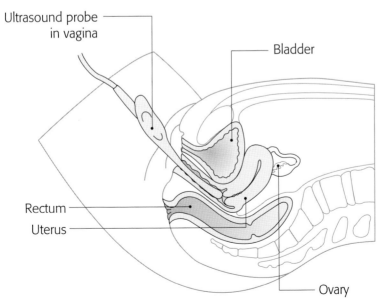

Hysteroscopy and curettage

- Hysteroscopy is a method of examining the uterus using a small telescope called a hysteroscope. It may be carried out under local anaesthetic in the out-patient clinic, or as a day-case procedure under general anaesthetic. It takes about 20 minutes.

- If you are awake, you will be asked to lie on your back with your legs in supports. The hysteroscope is passed through the vagina and cervix into the uterus. Gas or liquid is used to distend the uterus slightly to make the examination easier.

- A tissue sample or biopsy can be taken through some hysteroscopes. Alternatively, an endometrial biopsy device can be used, or the lining of the uterus can be scraped using an instrument called a curette (this is commonly known as a D & C). The tissue sample is sent for analysis.

- You may feel some discomfort similar to period pain for a few hours after hysteroscopy. You may also have a small amount of bleeding that lasts for 1–2 days.

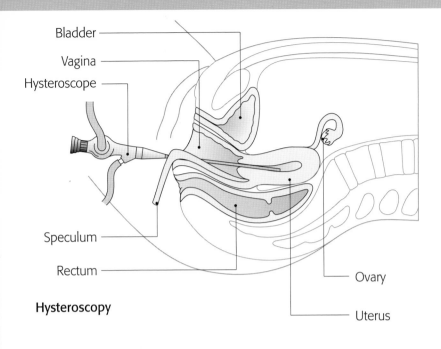

Bladder

Vagina

Hysteroscope

Speculum

Rectum

Ovary

Uterus

Hysteroscopy

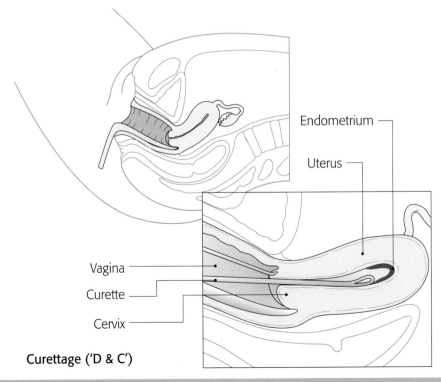

Endometrium

Uterus

Vagina

Curette

Cervix

Curettage ('D & C')

Hysterectomy for endometrial cancer

- The usual operation for endometrial cancer involves removing the uterus, cervix, both Fallopian tubes and ovaries. The procedure is called a total abdominal hysterectomy and bilateral salpingo-oophorectomy (TAH & BSO for short).

- Sometimes it is also necessary to remove the fat 'apron' in the abdomen (called the omentum), in a procedure called omentectomy. Similarly, the lymph glands in the pelvis may be removed.

- The operation is carried out under general anaesthetic, usually through a vertical (midline) or transverse (bikini-line) incision. A catheter may be passed up the urethra into the bladder to drain off the urine, and another tube may be inserted into the abdomen or vagina to drain any bleeding in the pelvis. These tubes may be left in place for 1–2 days.

- Sometimes, the hysterectomy is performed using keyhole surgery. A narrow telescope called a laparoscope is inserted through a small cut in the belly button. Keyhole surgery instruments are inserted into the abdomen through other small cuts in the abdominal wall. The laparoscope is used to perform the early steps of the hysterectomy, and the organs are finally removed through the vagina. Lymph glands in the pelvis can also be removed using the laparoscope.

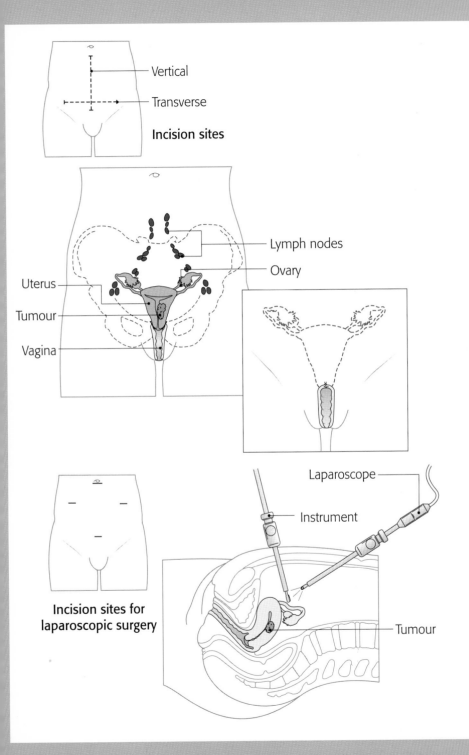

Vertical

Transverse

Incision sites

Lymph nodes

Ovary

Uterus

Tumour

Vagina

Laparoscope

Instrument

Incision sites for laparoscopic surgery

Tumour

VIN and vulval cancer

- Many conditions cause vulval itch, or pruritus. Changes in the vulval skin may be noticeable, but this does not necessarily indicate cancer.

- One cause of vulval itching is lichen sclerosis. This is a distressing condition that affects mainly elderly women. Although harmless in itself, women with lichen sclerosis have an increased risk of developing vulval cancer.

- Vulval intraepithelial neoplasia (VIN for short) is a pre-cancerous condition, and is associated with infection with a virus called the wart virus. VIN is not a cancer but it means that the cells are abnormal and have the potential to become cancerous.

- It is often not possible to distinguish between a non-cancerous condition and early cancer by appearance alone. VIN and vulval cancer may cause no symptoms, and VIN may appear normal to the naked eye.

- Vulval cancer spreads directly into the tissues next to the vulva, including the vagina, urethra, bladder and anus. Early spread or metastasis occurs through the lymph fluid channels into the lymph glands in the groin, and then to the lymph glands in the pelvis. Less commonly, metastasis occurs through the bloodstream, causing tumours to grow in distant sites such as the lungs and brain.

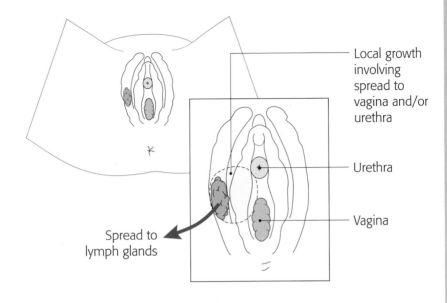

Local growth involving spread to vagina and/or urethra

Urethra

Vagina

Spread to lymph glands

Early spread to lymph nodes

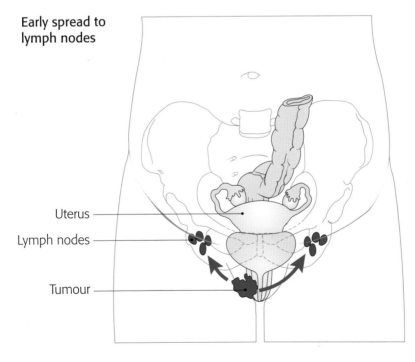

Uterus

Lymph nodes

Tumour

Vulval biopsy and treatment of VIN

- To diagnose vulval intraepithelial neoplasia (VIN for short), the vulva is examined in a procedure called vulvoscopy. A special microscope called a colposcope is usually used. Vulvoscopy is a painless, out-patient procedure. You will be asked to lie on your back with your legs in supports.

- Dilute acetic acid may be painted onto your vulva to show up any abnormal cells. This is not painful, but may cause mild irritation.

- Samples of vulval tissue, called vulval biopsies, may be removed for examination in the laboratory. These are taken either after numbing the area with local anaesthetic, or under a general anaesthetic. Your doctor may take several small circular punch biopsies (tiny circular samples of skin), or remove a larger piece of tissue (called an excision biopsy). You will probably need a few stitches after an excision biopsy, and these will leave a small scar.

- If you have VIN, the abnormal cells may be removed, or sometimes destroyed using a laser. This is usually carried out under general anaesthetic. You will be given painkillers and possibly also a local anaesthetic jelly to use for a few days after treatment.

- After VIN has been diagnosed, you will require regular vulvoscopy. An alternative way of managing this condition is to remove only areas that appear to be progressing towards early cancer. This may save unnecessary surgery.

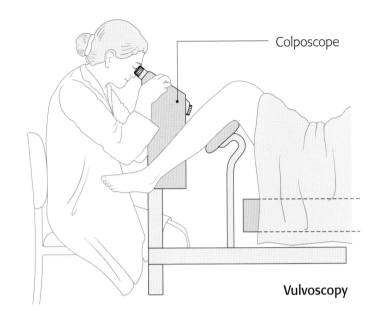

Colposcope

Vulvoscopy

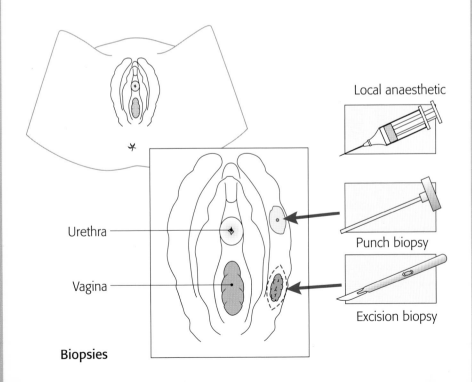

Local anaesthetic

Punch biopsy

Excision biopsy

Urethra

Vagina

Biopsies

Wide local excision, radical vulvectomy and groin node dissection

- If you have a small vulval cancer, it may be removed under general anaesthetic in a procedure called wide local excision. A small amount of normal surrounding tissue is also removed. Unless the cancer is at a very early stage, the lymph glands in one or both groins are also removed.

- You may be monitored with vulvoscopy up to four times a year to check that the cancer has not returned.

- If the cancer is more advanced, an operation called radical vulvectomy and groin node dissection is usually required. This involves removing the entire vulva and the lymph glands in the groins. If necessary, the lower part of the urethra can be removed without affecting bladder function. The skin with the pubic hair is not normally removed.

- The operation is carried out under general anaesthetic, usually through separate cuts in the groins and around the vulva. The skin at the bottom of the vagina is stitched directly to the skin outside of the vulva. Tubes drain lymph fluid from the groin wounds for up to 10 days after surgery.

- Depending on the pathology report, you may require radiotherapy after the wounds have healed. You will be seen regularly at the clinic for at least 5–10 years. Penetrative sex is usually, but not always, possible after a radical vulvectomy. If not, reconstructive surgery may be possible at a later date.

22

Wide local excision

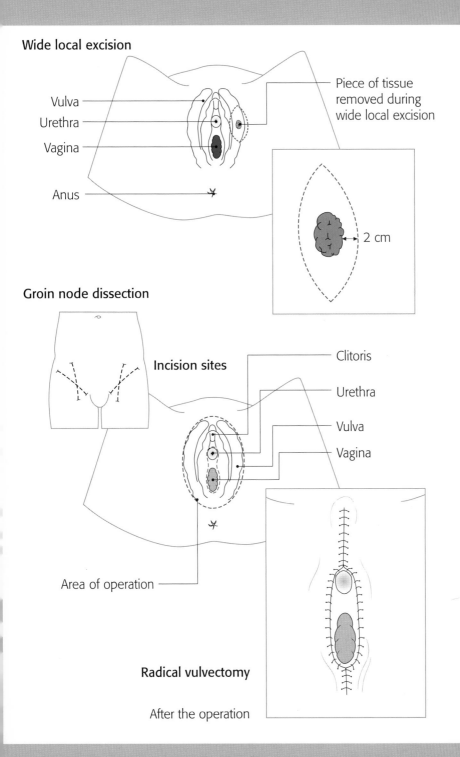

Vulva

Urethra

Vagina

Anus

Piece of tissue removed during wide local excision

2 cm

Groin node dissection

Incision sites

Clitoris

Urethra

Vulva

Vagina

Area of operation

Radical vulvectomy

After the operation

GTD and evacuation of the uterus

- Gestational trophoblastic disease (GTD for short) describes a range of conditions. At one end is the benign (non-cancerous) condition known as hydatidiform mole. At the other end is malignant (cancerous) choriocarcinoma. GTD is related to pregnancy, and occurs when the tissue that forms the placenta develops abnormally.

- Hydatidiform moles may be described as 'partial' or 'complete', depending on the tissue involved. Occasionally, a complete mole can develop into a choriocarcinoma.

- The treatment for hydatidiform mole is evacuation of the uterus. The pregnancy will not develop normally and must be removed to settle bleeding and enable the uterus to return to normal. Evacuation is carried out using a suction device under general anaesthetic, and takes about 10–15 minutes. You will normally be able to go home the next day. The diagnosis cannot be confirmed until the pathology result is known.

- After the operation, you will have regular urine tests to check that your pregnancy hormones are returning to normal levels. Do not take the contraceptive pill until this has happened, and wait for at least another 6 months before becoming pregnant again.

- If you need further treatment, or if you have a choriocarcinoma, you will be given chemotherapy, which is treatment with drugs that attack the abnormal cells. Most women are still able to become pregnant after chemotherapy. The risk of GTD occurring in the next pregnancy is increased, but is still small (about 1 in 100).

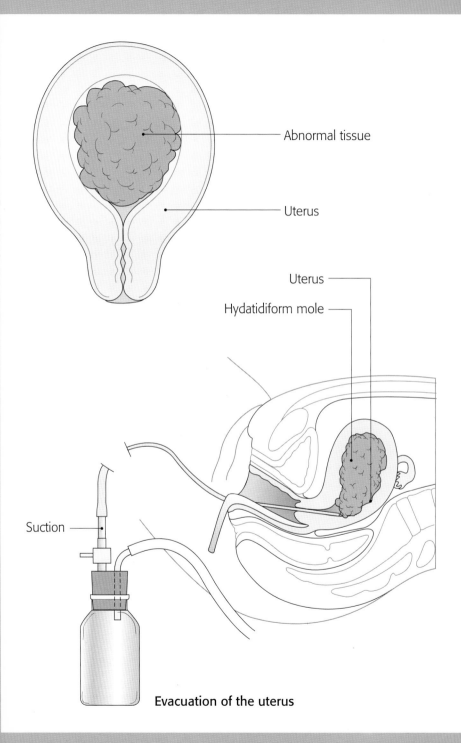

Abnormal tissue

Uterus

Uterus

Hydatidiform mole

Suction

Evacuation of the uterus

Radiotherapy

- Radiotherapy (X-ray treatment) can be used as either the main treatment for some cancers, or in addition to surgery and chemotherapy. It can also be used to treat cancer that has returned after treatment.

- A radiotherapist will first assess the area that needs radiotherapy, which is called the 'field', and calculate the dose and number of visits that you need.

- The two main types of radiotherapy are called external-beam radiotherapy and brachytherapy. With external-beam radiotherapy, an X-ray beam is directed at the area with the cancer, while brachytherapy involves leaving an X-ray-emitting device in the uterus or vagina. This is usually inserted under a general anaesthetic, and it may be left in place for up to a day, depending on the type of device used.

- You may have skin rashes, diarrhoea, bladder irritation, tiredness and flu-like symptoms during and straight after treatment. Many of these can be relieved with medical treatments, although bladder or bowel irritation may persist for months or become permanent. In young women, the ovaries may stop making hormones, and hormone-replacement therapy (HRT) may be needed on a long-term basis.

- A very uncommon but serious possible side-effect is fistula formation, where an opening forms between either the bowel or urinary system and the vagina. An operation is usually required to overcome this problem.

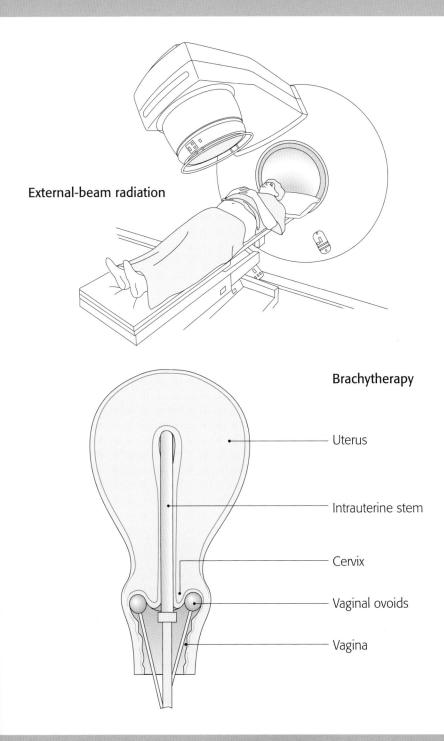

External-beam radiation

Brachytherapy

Uterus

Intrauterine stem

Cervix

Vaginal ovoids

Vagina

Chemotherapy

- Chemotherapy is treatment with drugs that destroy cancer cells. Cancer cells that remain after surgery or those that have spread to distant sites can be treated with chemotherapy. However, some normal body cells are also affected, causing side-effects.

- Some chemotherapy causes sickness, though modern anti-sickness drugs can reduce this. Some, but not all, forms of chemotherapy cause hair loss. Your doctor will explain the particular side-effects that your treatment may cause and will perform blood tests before giving each course of treatment.

- The choice of drugs used depends on the type of cancer, your health and possibly your age. Most chemotherapy uses a combination of drugs to maximize effectiveness and minimize side-effects. You will be given chemotherapy drugs according to a certain timetable. For example, they might be given once every 3 weeks, over 15 weeks. This allows your body, especially your blood cells, to recover between each treatment. Most treatments are given on an out-patient basis.

- Usually, chemotherapy drugs are given through a drip or by injection into a plastic tube or cannula inserted into a vein in the arm, though some can be given as tablets.

- For certain types of cancer, high-dose hormone treatment may slow the growth of the cancer, or even shrink it. Hormone therapy generally has fewer side-effects than chemotherapy.

Chemotherapy

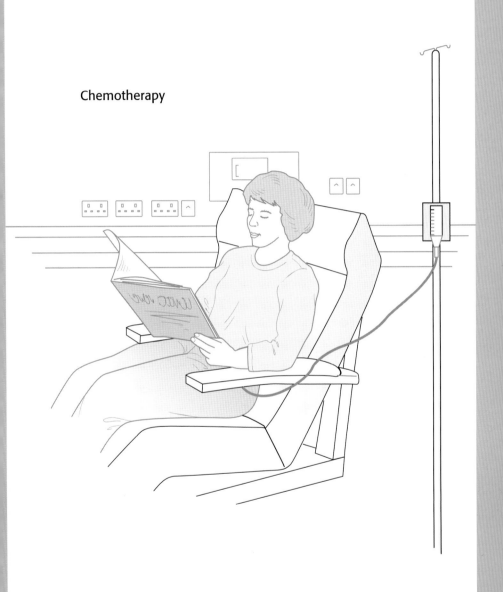

Exenteration surgery

- A return or recurrence of cancer after treatment does not necessarily mean that the cancer has become incurable, but further surgery called exenteration surgery may be needed. The aim is to try and cure the cancer, and this surgery is only considered if the cancer has not spread elsewhere in the body. It involves removing some or all of the pelvic organs that were left in place after your first operation.

- Total exenteration involves removal of the bladder and surrounding tissues including the urethra, the lower parts of the bowel (anus and rectum), vulva and vagina. Anterior exenteration surgery involves removal of the bladder but not the anus and rectum, while posterior exenteration involves removal of the anus and rectum but not the bladder. A procedure called supralevator exenteration preserves the tissues below the floor of the pelvis, in particular the vulva and the lower vagina.

- These operations are carried out under general anaesthetic, through incisions made in the abdomen and between the legs. Supralevator exenteration requires an abdominal incision only.

- Depending on the organs that are removed, you will need a urinary diversion for urine and/or a colostomy for faeces. These involve making one or more openings (stoma) in the abdominal wall so that the urine and/or contents of the bowel can be collected in a bag or bags outside the body.

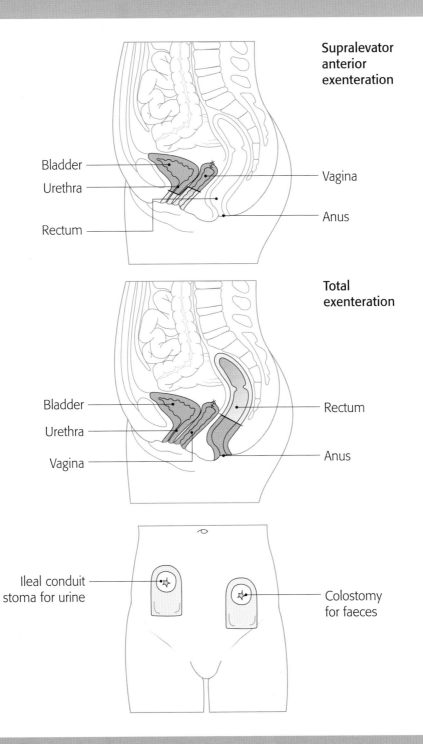

Supralevator anterior exenteration

Bladder

Urethra

Rectum

Vagina

Anus

Total exenteration

Bladder

Urethra

Vagina

Rectum

Anus

Ileal conduit stoma for urine

Colostomy for faeces

Fistulae

- A ureterovaginal fistula is an opening between one of the ureters and the vagina. It usually results from surgery and it causes urine to leak through the vagina. Initially it may be treated by passing a tube, or stent, into the ureter. If it does not close over, it is repaired through the abdomen by joining the healthy ureter above the fistula to the bladder.

- A vesicovaginal fistula is an opening between the bladder and the vagina, and causes urine to leak from the vagina. It can occur as a result of tumour invasion, after surgery or, particularly, after radiotherapy. It may be repaired through the vagina or by a cut in the abdomen, and the vagina may need to be closed. A piece of tissue may be removed from the labia or from inside the abdomen, and used to separate the bladder and vagina to prevent the fistula from returning. If the fistula is caused by tumour recurrence, repair is not possible, but incontinence can be cured by a urinary diversion. This involves making an opening in the abdominal wall so that the urine can be collected in a bag outside the body.

- A rectovaginal fistula is an opening between the rectum, which is the bottom part of the large bowel, and the vagina. As a result, the contents of the bowel can pass out of the vagina, causing a distressing discharge. Repair may be possible, but if not, a colostomy will overcome the problem. This involves making an opening in the abdomen so that the contents of the bowel can be collected outside the body in a stoma bag.

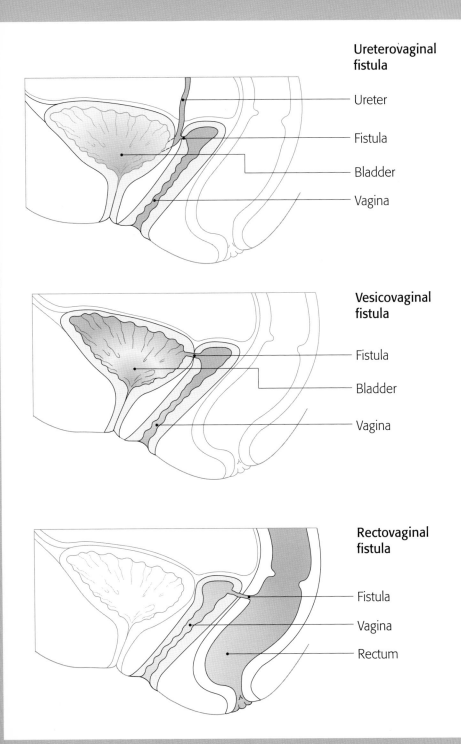

27

Ureterovaginal fistula

— Ureter

— Fistula

— Bladder

— Vagina

Vesicovaginal fistula

— Fistula

— Bladder

— Vagina

Rectovaginal fistula

— Fistula

— Vagina

— Rectum

Urinary diversion, ileostomy and colostomy

- If your bladder and urethra have to be removed in an exenteration procedure, or you have a urinary fistula that cannot be closed, your surgeon will make a passage (called a conduit) from a section of your small bowel. The flow of urine is redirected from the kidney so that it drains through this passage. An opening called a stoma is made in the abdominal wall, and the urine drains continuously into a bag that is worn on the abdomen. Sometimes 'continent' urinary diversions can be made. These collect urine like a bladder behind the abdominal wall and are emptied by passing a catheter into the stoma.

- If some of your bowel has been removed, or you have a bowel blockage or rectovaginal fistula, you may need an ileostomy or a colostomy. The stoma is made in the abdominal wall, and this allows the contents of the bowel to be collected in a bag that is worn on the abdomen. Depending on your health, the reason that the stoma was made and what part of the bowel has been removed, you may be able to have the ileostomy or colostomy closed some months later. However, most stomas created for patients with gynaecological cancer are permanent.

- If you have urinary diversion and/or an ileostomy or colostomy, you will be given counselling before the operation, and help afterwards until you are able to manage the stoma(s) yourself.

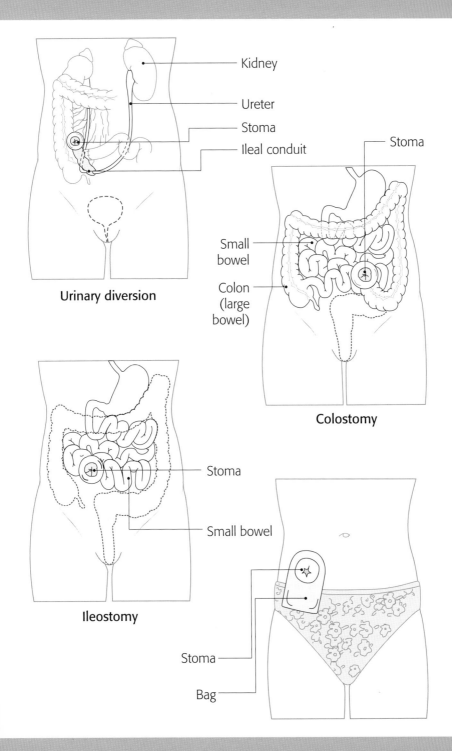

28

Kidney

Ureter

Stoma

Ileal conduit

Stoma

Small bowel

Colon (large bowel)

Urinary diversion

Colostomy

Stoma

Small bowel

Ileostomy

Stoma

Bag

Nephrostomy and ureteric stents

- The ureter connects the kidney with the bladder, and can become blocked if the cancer is pressing on it. Severe cramping pain can occur and the kidney can stop working altogether if the urine flow is not restored. Nephrostomy and ureteric stenting are techniques that can overcome this type of blockage.

- With a nephrostomy, a tube is inserted through the skin of the back into the kidney, so that the urine can be drained and collected in a bag. The procedure is carried out under local anaesthetic, and ultrasound or X-rays are used for guidance.

- A ureteric stent is a narrow flexible plastic tube that can be passed along the inside of a ureter to allow the kidney to drain normally.

- A retrograde ureteric stent is inserted upwards from the bladder using a narrow telescope, called a cystoscope, that is inserted through the urethra. The stent is inserted under a general anaesthetic and, once in place, extends from the kidney down to the bladder.

- An antegrade stent is inserted through a nephrostomy tube and then down the ureter and into the bladder.

- Stents are also placed into ureters to help them heal after operations such as ureteric fistula repairs and urinary diversions. You will probably be given antibiotics to take while you have a ureteric stent in place. Stents can easily be removed in a short, 20-minute procedure under a general anaesthetic.

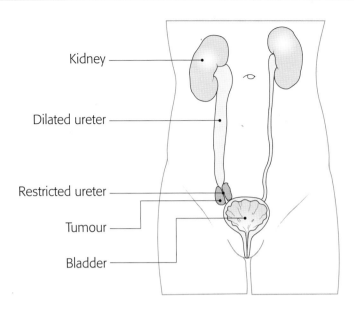

29

Kidney

Dilated ureter

Restricted ureter

Tumour

Bladder

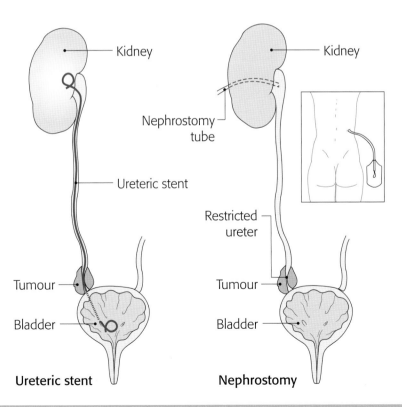

Kidney

Kidney

Nephrostomy tube

Ureteric stent

Restricted ureter

Tumour

Tumour

Bladder

Bladder

Ureteric stent

Nephrostomy

Intestinal obstruction

- Tumours that press on or spread to the bowel can cause intestinal obstruction. The symptoms depend on where the blockage is, but may include nausea, cramping pain, vomiting and abdominal swelling. Bowel obstruction is a common problem for women with advanced ovarian cancer.

- To relieve the condition at first, you may be given fluids by intravenous drip. The build up of stomach and bowel contents above the obstruction can be reduced using gentle suction through a nasogastric tube, which is passed through the nose into the stomach.

- It may be possible to remove the blocked part of bowel surgically, or to bypass it by joining one part of the bowel to another. Alternatively, an obstruction may be bypassed with an ileostomy or colostomy, which involves making an opening or stoma in the wall of the abdomen. The contents of the bowel can then be collected in a bag worn outside the abdomen.

- Chemotherapy, which involves using drugs to attack the cancer cells, can sometimes gradually shrink the tumour and relieve the blockage.

- Often it is not possible to remove or shrink the tumour, so the effects of the obstruction have to be managed with medications. You may be given fluid through a fine plastic tube that is inserted under the skin. You may be able to continue to drink small amounts of high-protein and high-calorie drinks.

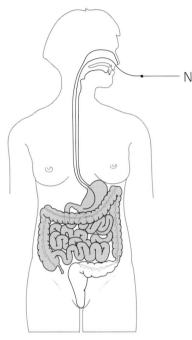

30

Nasogastric tube

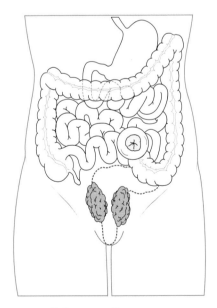

Colostomy for tumour
blocking rectum

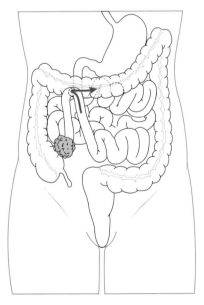

Anastomosis for
ileocaecal obstruction

Ascites and pleural effusion

- Fluid can accumulate in the abdomen or chest as a side-effect of cancer. Fluid in the abdomen is called ascites, while that in the chest is called a pleural effusion. These problems are common in women with ovarian cancer.

- A pleural effusion can make breathing difficult by compressing the lungs as it accumulates. Ascites can be uncomfortable and can also make breathing difficult.

- The fluid can be removed using a syringe or by inserting a drain, after the area has been numbed with local anaesthetic. The procedure can be repeated if more fluid builds up. Ascites is not usually removed before you have surgery, unless you are very uncomfortable. It will be taken away using a suction tube at the start of the operation.

- Treatment of the cancer cells using surgery and, particularly, chemotherapy may reduce the rate at which fluid builds up. It may cause the ascites and/or pleural effusion to disappear.

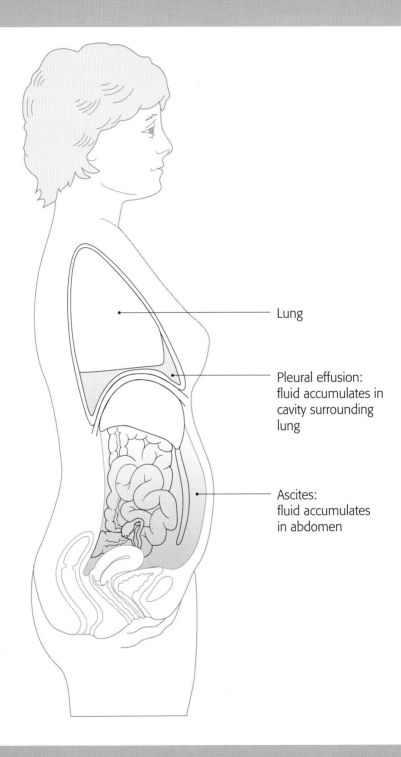

31

Lung

Pleural effusion:
fluid accumulates in
cavity surrounding
lung

Ascites:
fluid accumulates
in abdomen

Pain relief

- Pain in terminal cancer is best treated by analgesics, which are painkillers, together with strategies to relieve the specific causes of the pain.

- Cramping pain can occur if you have a blockage in, for example, your bowel. Antispasmodic drugs can give immediate relief, and surgical procedures can sometimes be used to overcome the blockage, depending on where it is.

- Tumours can cause pressure on the nerves, causing severe stabbing or burning pains. As well as analgesics, several other types of medication are good at easing this type of pain. Special injections, including local anaesthetics, can act as nerve blocks, and injections of a strong analgesic into the space around the spinal cord can also be effective.

- The type and dose of painkiller are adjusted to ensure that your pain is relieved. Narcotics are the strongest painkillers and are extremely effective. Side-effects such as constipation and, possibly, nausea require treatment with other medicines. If drowsiness becomes a problem, the dose can be adjusted. Narcotics can be given by a needle under the skin, skin patches, suppositories, tablets or syrup, with extra doses available to 'top up' the pain relief when required.

- Alternative therapies, such as acupuncture, aromatherapy, massage, hypnosis and meditation, are effective in relieving pain or the side-effects of drug treatments for some terminally ill cancer patients.

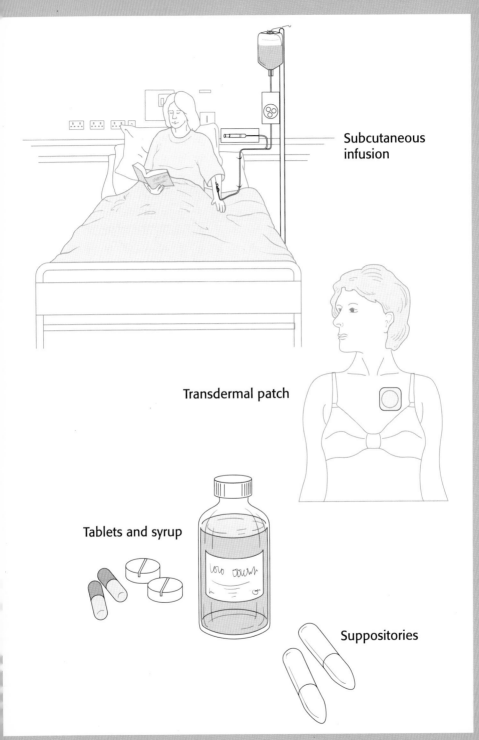

32

Subcutaneous
infusion

Transdermal patch

Tablets and syrup

Suppositories

Mail order

This *Patient Pictures* book is one of a rapidly growing series.

Current titles include:
- *Bladder disorders*
- *Cardiology*
- *Fertility*
- *Gastroenterology*
- *Genitourinary medicine*
- *Gynaecology (second edition)*
- *HIV medicine*
- *Prostatic diseases and their treatments (second edition)*
- *Respiratory diseases*
- *Rheumatology (second edition)*
- *Urological surgery*

For an up-to-date list of *Health Press* titles or to order, simply phone or fax:

Tel: +44 (0)1235 523233
Fax: +44 (0)1235 523238

Or why not visit our website
www.patientpictures.com